T0144719

THE
CHELATION
CONTROVERSY

HOW TO SAFELY DETOXIFY YOUR BODY AND IMPROVE YOUR HEALTH AND WELL-BEING

Gregory Pouls, D.C., F.I.C.N.,
and Maile Pouls, Ph.D.

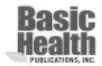

**Basic
Health**
PUBLICATIONS, INC.

The information contained in this book is based upon the research and personal and professional experiences of the authors. It is not intended as a substitute for consulting with your physician or other healthcare provider. Any attempt to diagnose and treat an illness should be done under the direction of a healthcare professional.

The publisher does not advocate the use of any particular healthcare protocol but believes the information in this book should be available to the public. The publisher and authors are not responsible for any adverse effects or consequences resulting from the use of the suggestions, preparations, or procedures discussed in this book. Should the reader have any questions concerning the appropriateness of any procedures or preparation mentioned, the authors and the publisher strongly suggest consulting a professional healthcare advisor.

Editor: Jane E. Morrill
Typesetter: Gary A. Rosenberg
Series Cover Designer: Mike Stromberg

Basic Health Guides are published by
Basic Health Publications, Inc.

ISBN: 978-1-59120-056-7 (Pbk.)
ISBN: 978-1-68162-795-3 (Hardcover)

Contents

"Drs. Gregory and Maile Pouls have written an informative, basic, and interesting account of the chelation controversy. This book is a great place to start for those exploring a detoxification program that will be instrumental to understanding the great new emerging field of Metabolic Cardiology."

—Dr. Stephen T. Sinatra

Stephen T. Sinatra, M.D., F.A.C.C., F.A.C.N., is one of America's most respected and recognized natural-minded cardiologists. A board-certified cardiologist and certified psychotherapist, Dr. Sinatra has more than twenty-five years of experience helping patients prevent and reverse heart disease.

Introduction

The past sixty years have seen a chemical revolution around the world. Our bodies and personal environments have been altered by the gradual accumulation of heavy metals and synthetic (human-made) chemicals. Each day, we are all exposed to small amounts of thousands of recently created chemicals that our bodies must learn to adapt to and cope with.

The health effects from massive exposure to many of these chemicals and metals have been known for years. However, long-term chronic exposure to small amounts of heavy metals and toxic chemicals that accumulate in our tissues contributes to cancer, heart disease, reproductive dysfunction, arthritis, neurological conditions (including Alzheimer's disease, Parkinson's disease, and dementia), dysfunction of the endocrine glands (hormone-producing glands), allergies, fatigue, immune-system dysfunction, skin conditions, and more. Many of these conditions, considered rare 100 years ago, are now common, even expected, in adults living in the urban and agricultural regions of America. Worse, many of these degenerative diseases are now appearing in children and adolescents.

The human body is equipped with numerous detoxification pathways—primarily the colon, liver, kidneys, lungs, and skin. Eventually, however, the body accumulates toxins faster than it can eliminate them, so it stores them in the liver and other fatty tissues, such as the brain and endocrine glands, where they initiate degenerative processes.

Whether you live in the city or the country—especially in agricultural areas—everyone is exposed to heavy metals and oxidizing chemicals on a daily basis. Exposure comes primarily from contaminants in our air, food, and water. (To find out how toxic your neighborhood is, visit www.scorecard.org and enter your zip code in the "Find Your Community" box. You will get a detailed summary of the chemical hazards in your community.) You can limit further exposure by using air and water filters in your home and by eating organic foods, but don't think you're safe because you live in the country and eat organic. (To learn about organic farming and the chemicals and metals commonly found in commercially grown fruits and vegetables, see www.organicconsumers.org/toxiclink.html.)

More than 6 *billion* pounds of chemical toxins are released into American environments every year. Most Americans believe that the Environmental Protection Agency (EPA) and the Food and Drug Administration (FDA) have set industry standards for the release of toxins and limits for safe exposure to them. We have been taught that most chemicals are safe. Unfortunately, none of this is true. Of the more than 75,000 chemicals registered with the EPA, relatively few have been thoroughly tested to determine their effects on human health, and only about 600 must be reported to the EPA's Toxic Release Inventory. Many chemicals that are produced in vast quantities have never been studied at all, and studies showing the health effects of various chemicals combined together are almost nonexistent. Case in point:

- More than 3,000 chemicals are added to our food supplies.

- 700 chemicals have been found in "tap" water.

- 400 chemicals have been identified in human breast milk, tissues, and urine.

- 500 chemicals are routinely found under kitchen and laundry-room sinks. With thousands of cleaning, daily-use, and personal-care products, information about potentially harmful chemicals isn't always listed on the label. If it is, it's often shown in terms that only a Ph.D. chemist could understand. Full disclosure may be hidden in "proprietary formulas" or "inert ingredients."

- The average American home contains about 100 pounds of hazardous chemicals and waste.[1]

We have to learn how to reduce or eliminate further exposure and to safely rid our bodies of accumulated stored chemicals and metals. Intravenous (IV) and oral chelation (pronounced "key-LAY-shun") therapies allow us to safely and effectively detoxify our bodies of metals and chemicals, while nutritionally supporting our organs, glands, and tissues.

WHAT IS CHELATION?

The word "chelation" comes from the Greek word "chele," which means "claw." Chelating agents are substances that grab on to, or chemically bond with, minerals and metals in the body. A chelating agent encircles a mineral or metal ion and carries it from the body via the urine or feces.

The chelation process is common in nature. The process of digesting and absorbing nutrients from our food uses chelation between amino acids (building blocks of protein) and minerals to deliver nutrients to specific cells or tissues in the body. The creation and function of enzymes (biological catalysts) depends on chelation, as does the creation of hormones (biochemical messengers).

Both IV and oral chelation have benefits and drawbacks. Different doctors and researchers may tell you that they both work, that only one works, or that neither works. It can be very confusing.

IV chelation therapy involves the injection of a synthetic amino acid, usually ethylenediaminetetraacetic acid (EDTA), to bond with and eliminate heavy metals, chemical toxins, mineral deposits, fatty plaques, and other unwanted substances from the body. EDTA has been widely studied and is effective against most metals; however, it has a limited ability to chelate mercury. Another chemical chelating agent, dimercaptopropanesulfonic acid (DMPS), although not approved by the FDA, has been used intravenously to remove mercury. At the end of your IV chelation treatment you should be provided with "replacement nutrients" to replace the healthy metals and minerals that are removed along with the unhealthy metals and toxins during treatment.

Some nutritionally oriented medical doctors also provide nutrient-based IV treatments to enhance the chelation process or to address specific health conditions. Oral chelation therapy involves ingesting nutritional supplements and other natural and synthetic substances (oral EDTA, for example) that have chelating abilities. Amino acids, antioxidant nutrients, herbs, minerals, phytonutrients ("phyto" means "plant"), and vitamins are added to enhance the benefits of oral chelation.

1. The Big Six Heavy Metals

Heavy metals are like the bullies in the schoolyard; they are bigger and heavier than the smaller ones and like to push them out of line. That's how heavy metals compete for cell-binding sites, too. However, having a body that is nutritionally sufficient, with minerals and beneficial metals already filling its cell-binding sites, helps to protect you from further heavy-metal buildup.

The most prevalent heavy metals are aluminum, arsenic, cadmium, lead, mercury, and nickel. Why are they called "heavy" metals? Because they have a higher molecular weight than most substances, including minerals.

1. ALUMINUM	
Sources of exposure	Aluminum cookware, aluminum foil, antacids, anti-perspirants, baking powder (aluminum-containing), buffered aspirin, canned acidic foods, food additives, lipstick, medications and drugs (antidiarrhea agents, hemorrhoid medications, vaginal douches), processed cheese, softened water, and tap water.
Target tissues	Bones, brain, kidneys, and stomach.
Signs and symptoms	Colic, dementia, esophagitis, gastroenteritis, kidney damage, liver dysfunction, loss of appetite, loss of balance, muscle pain, psychosis, shortness of breath, and weakness.
Protective nutritional substances	Magnesium.

Recent studies suggest that aluminum also contributes to neurological disorders such as Alzheimer's disease, Parkinson's disease, and senile and presenile dementia, clumsiness of movements, staggering when walking, and the inability to pronounce words correctly. Behavioral difficulties among schoolchildren also show a direct correlation with elevated levels of aluminum and other heavy metals. Toxic levels of aluminum have been found in many neurological conditions.

2. ARSENIC	
Sources of exposure	Air pollution, antibiotics in commercial livestock, certain marine plants, chemical processing, coal-fired power plants, defoliants, drying agents for cotton, fish, herbicides, insecticides, meats (commercially raised cattle, poultry), metal-ore smelting, pesticides, seafood (fish, mussels, oysters), specialty glass, tap water, and wood preservatives.
Target tissues	Most organs, especially in the gastrointestinal system, lungs, and skin.
Signs and symptoms	Abdominal pain, burning of the mouth and throat, cancer (especially lung, skin), coma, diarrhea, nausea, neuritis, peripheral vascular problems, skin lesions, and vascular collapse.
Protective nutritional substances	Amino acids containing sulfur, calcium, iodine, selenium, vitamin C, and zinc.

The greatest dangers from chronic arsenic exposure are lung and skin cancers and gradual poisoning, most often from living near metal-smelting plants or arsenic factories.

3. CADMIUM	
Sources of exposure	Air pollution, art supplies, bonemeal, coffee, crab, flounder, fruits, fresh-water fish, fungicides, grains, highway dusts, incinerators, meats (kidneys, liver, poultry), mining, mussels, nickel-cadmium batteries, oxide dusts, oysters, paints, phosphate fertilizers, power plants, refined foods, scallops, sewage sludge, smelting plants, softened water, tobacco smoke, vegetables from cadmium-laden soil, and welding fumes.
Target tissues	Appetite and pain centers in the brain, brain, heart and blood vessels, kidneys, and lungs.

Signs and symptoms	Anemia, depressed immune-system response, dry and scaly skin, emphysema, fatigue, hair loss, heart disease, hypertension, joint pain, kidney stones or damage, liver dysfunction or damage, loss of appetite, loss of sense of smell, lung cancer, pain in the back and legs, and yellow teeth.
Protective nutritional substances	Amino acids containing sulfur, calcium, vitamin C, and zinc.

Current studies are trying to determine whether adequate calcium, protein (amino acids), vitamin C, and zinc can prevent or lessen cadmium-induced bone and kidney damage.

4. LEAD

Sources of exposure	Air pollution, ammunition, auto exhaust, bathtubs (cast iron, porcelain, steel), batteries, canned foods, ceramics, chemical fertilizers, colored ads, cosmetics, dolomite, dust, foods grown near industrial areas, gasoline, hair dyes and rinses, leaded glass, newsprint, paints, pesticides, pewter, pottery, rubber toys, soft coal, soil, solder, tap water, tobacco smoke, and vinyl miniblinds.
Target tissues	Bones, brain, heart, kidneys, liver, nervous system, and pancreas.
Signs and symptoms	Abdominal pain, anemia, anorexia, anxiety, bone pain, brain damage, confusion, constipation, convulsions, dizziness, drowsiness, fatigue, headaches, hypertension, inability to concentrate, indigestion, irritability, loss of appetite, loss of muscle coordination, memory difficulties, miscarriage, muscle pain, pallor, tremors, vomiting, and weakness.
Protective nutritional substances	Amino acids containing sulfur, calcium, iron, vitamin C, vitamin E, and zinc.

A known neurotoxin that kills brain cells, excessive levels of lead in children's blood have been linked to learning disabilities, attention deficit disorder (ADD), attention deficit hyperactivity disorder (ADHD), reduced intelligence test scores, and lower achievement in school. The greatest risk of lead poisoning, even with only minute or short-term exposure, is to infants, young children, and pregnant women.

5. MERCURY	
Sources of exposure	Air pollution, batteries, cosmetics, dental amalgams, diuretics (mercurial), electrical devices and relays, explosives, fluorescent lights, freshwater fish (especially large bass, pike, and trout), fungicides, grains, insecticides, mining, paints, pesticides, petroleum products, saltwater fish (especially large halibut, shrimp, snapper, and swordfish), shellfish, and tap water.
Target tissues	Appetite and pain centers in the brain, cell membranes, kidneys, and nervous system (central and peripheral).
Signs and symptoms	Abnormal nervous and physical development (fetal and childhood), anemia, anorexia, anxiety, blindness, blood changes, blue line on gums, colitis, depression, dermatitis, difficulty chewing and swallowing, dizziness, drowsiness, emotional instability, excessive salivation, fatigue, fever, hallucinations, headache, hearing loss, hypertension, inflamed gums, insomnia, kidney damage or failure, loss of appetite and sense of smell, loss of muscle coordination, memory loss, metallic taste in mouth, nerve damage, numbness, psychosis, stomatitis, tremors, vision impairment, vomiting, weakness, and weight loss.
Protective nutritional substances	Amino acids (containing sulfur), pectin (alginate), selenium, and vitamin C.

The primary source of exposure to mercury is "silver" dental fillings (approximately 50 percent mercury when placed). They release microscopic particles and mercury vapors every time a person chews. The vapors are inhaled while particles are absorbed by tooth roots, mucous membranes of the mouth and gums, and the stomach lining.

More than 225 million Americans have mercury-amalgam fillings in their teeth. Probably the greatest short-term exposure to mercury vapors occurs while having "old" silver/mercury amalgam dental fillings removed. The process of cutting the "old" filling into pieces for removal releases massive amounts of mercury vapor into the patient's (and dentist's) air space. For this reason, if you are considering having your "old" silver/mercury amalgam fillings removed, we urge you to seek assistance from a biological dentist. Biological dentists do not use mercury in their practices and are trained to safely remove "old" silver/ mercury amalgam fillings, without exposing the patient to mercury vapors. To locate a biological dentist in your area, please visit www.talk international.com. Scroll down the left margin toolbar to Mercury Free & Biological Dental Dentistry. Or visit www.medical-library.net/ and click on Click Here to Find a Dentist and under "Specialties" select Biological and Mercury Free Dentistry.

In a person with mercury-based dental filings, the range of mercury-vapor levels can range from 20–400 micrograms per cubic meter (mcg/m^3), continuous exposure.

The following are current mercury exposure limits, according to various U.S. governmental health agencies:

• **American Conference of Governmental Industrial Hygienists (ACGIH)** does not consider mercury vapor a human carcinogen; however, it has set a mercury-vapor threshold limit value (TLV) of 0.025 mg/m^3 for a normal eight-hour workday and a forty-hour work week. The ACGIH also notes that human skin is an important route into the body for mercury vapors.

• **Environmental Protection Agency (EPA)** reference dose (RfD) for chronic oral (mercury vapor) exposure is not available at this time (www.epa.gov/iris/subst/0370.htm); EPA RfD for chronic oral (inorganic mercuric chloride) exposure limit: 0.0003 mg/kg/day; EPA RfD for chronic oral (methylmercury) exposure limit: 0.0001 mg/kg/day. EPA reference concentration for chronic inhalation (elemental mercury) exposure—EPA LOAEL (lowest observed adverse effect level) is set at 0.025 mg/m^3 (converted to LOAEL of 0.009 mg/ m^3). The LOAEL is based on an eight-hour occupational exposure. LOAEL is a level that should not be considered safe for everyone. The "critical effects" from LOAEL exposure to chronic inhalation of elemental mercury include hand tremor, increases in memory disturbance, and slight subjective and objective evidence of autonomic (nervous system) dysfunction (www.epa.gov/iris/subst/0370.htm). According to the EPA and ATSDR (Agency for Toxic Substances and Disease Registry), the toxic metals arsenic, cadmium, lead, and mercury are all ranked in the top seven toxic substances having the greatest adverse health effects on the public based on current exposure levels in the United States.[1] The EPA reports that approximately one-fourth of all infants in America are exposed to dangerous mercury levels. It has set the limit for mercury in drinking water to 2 parts of mercury per billion parts of drinking water (2 ppb).

- **Food and Drug Administration (FDA)** has set a maximum allowable level of 1 part of methylmercury in a million parts of seafood (1 ppm), with a warning at 0.5 ppm.

  On March 19, 2004, the FDA and the EPA announced a consumer advisory on methylmercury in fish and shellfish. This advisory is aimed at reducing exposure to high levels of mercury in pregnant women, women who may become pregnant, nursing mothers, and young children. The advisory states, "women might wish to modify the amount and type of fish they consume if they are pregnant, planning to become pregnant, nursing, or feeding a young child." (To learn more, visit www.fda.gov/bbs/topics/news/2004/NEW01038.html.)

- **Occupational Safety and Health Administration (OSHA)** has set "ceiling" limits of 0.1 milligram of organic mercury per cubic meter of workplace air (0.1 mg/m^3) and 0.05 mg/m^3 of metallic mercury vapor for eight-hour shifts and forty-hour work weeks. A worker's exposure to mercury vapor shall at no time exceed this ceiling level.

- **National Institute for Occupational Safety and Health (NIOSH)** has set a recommended exposure limit (REL) for mercury vapor of 0.05 mg/m^3 for up to a ten-hour workday and a forty-hour work week. NIOSH also informs the public that mercury-vapor exposure to the eyes, mucous membranes, and skin are additional factors in assessing overall mercury exposure.

None of these figures addresses continuous exposure from internal mercury, such as exposure from silver/mercury dental fillings or from vaccines that contain thimerosal/mercury.

Mercury Exposure from Vaccines

Thimerosal is a form of organic mercury containing antibacterial and antifungal properties. It has been used as a preservative in vaccinations and pharmaceutical products for more than seventy years. Exposure to mercury from vaccines is now being linked to numerous adult immune and neurological health conditions such as Alzheimer's disease and Parkinson's disease, and many scientists, researchers, and doctors believe thimerosal/mercury exposure from vaccines is a key factor in the sudden "epidemic" of childhood conditions such as autism, ADD, ADHD, dyslexia, and numerous other learning and behavioral disabilities. How could this be possible? A vaccine containing 0.01% thimerosal as a preservative contains 50 micrograms of thimerosal, or approximately 25 micrograms of mercury, per 0.5 ml dose (www.fda.gov/cber/vaccine/thimerosal.htm#thi). Currently, thimerosal is being reduced or eliminated from some vaccines, but numerous "childhood" and flu vaccines still contain this highly toxic mercury compound.

The current Childhood and Adolescent Immunization Schedule—approved by the Advisory Committee on Immunization Practices (www.cd.gov/nip/acip), the American Academy of Pediatrics (www.aap.org), and the American Academy of Family Physicians (www.aafp.org)—recommends ten different vaccinations by the age of eighteen months. Based upon the FDA report above (25 micrograms of mercury per 0.5 ml vaccine dose), this means in the first eighteen months of life a child could receive approximately 250 micrograms of mercury along with their vaccines—far exceeding the safe limits set by any governmental organization. We find it interesting that the symptoms for autism and mercury poisoning in children are nearly identical.

On February 9, 2004, the National Autism Association released a report based upon the Centers for Disease Control (CDC) Vaccine Safety Datalink. Independent investigators who reviewed the CDC's data concluded, "children are 27 times more likely to develop autism after exposure to three thimerosal-containing vaccines (TCVs), than those who receive thimerosal-free versions." Soon after release, the CDC rejected and "pulled" the study, stating the data was flawed.

If you are considering vaccinating yourself or your children, we urge you to educate yourself about the potential risks associated with thimerosal and vaccines. Please visit www.know-vaccines.org/faq.html.

6. NICKEL	
Sources of exposure	Appliances, buttons, ceramics, cocoa, cold-wave hair permanents, cooking utensils, cosmetics, coins, dental materials, food (chocolate, hydrogenated oils, nuts, food grown near industrial areas), hair spray, industrial waste, jewelry, medical implants, metal refineries, metal tools, nickel-cadmium batteries, orthodontic appliances, shampoo, solid-waste incinerators, stainless-steel kitchen utensils, tap water, tobacco smoke, water faucets, water pipes, and zippers.
Target tissues	Areas of skin exposure, larynx (voice box), lungs, and nasal passages.
Signs and symptoms	Apathy, blue-colored lips, cancer (especially lung, nasal, larynx), contact dermatitis, diarrhea, dizziness, fever, gingivitis, headaches, insomnia, nausea, rapid heart rate, shortness of breath, skin rashes (blisters, itching, redness), stomatitis, and vomiting.
Protective nutritional substances	Vitamin C (ascorbic acid).[2]

The greatest dangers from chronic nickel exposure are lung, nasal, and larynx cancers, and gradual poisoning from accidental or chronic low-level exposure. The risk is greatest for those living near metal-smelting plants, solid-waste incinerators, or old nickel refineries.[3]

THE TOXIC LOAD

According to logic, once the potential harm from heavy metals is understood, their production and use in America and around the world should be phased out and their storage heavily regulated. However, except for lead, the use of which has been curtailed, logic has taken a backseat to profit.

Even if all heavy-metal production were to stop today, enough heavy metals have already been released into our environment to cause chronic poisoning and numerous neurological diseases for generations to come. There are presently 600,000 toxic-waste contamination sites in the United States alone, according to the Congressional Office of Technology Assessment. Of these, the EPA has proposed fewer than 900 for superfund cleanup; approximately 19,000 others are under review.

We must take measures to protect ourselves from the hazards of heavy metals, because our government is doing little to protect us. Conventional medicine contends that the only way we can deal with this problem is to avoid known sources. But heavy metals are so widespread that they're impossible to avoid. Fortunately, alternative medicine provides a way to rid our bodies of these harmful substances. Intravenous (IV) and oral chelation detoxification protocols and supportive nutritional therapies can remove heavy metals and chemical toxins from our bodies and reduce our toxic load.

2. Free Radicals, Oxidation, and Antioxidants

If you've ever seen a nail rusting on a fence post or a slice of apple turn brown from exposure to oxygen, you've seen oxidation in action. Oxidation involves the "burning" of substances with oxygen; for example, bleach and hydrogen peroxide work by oxidation. Both animals and humans need oxygen to live; however, in certain instances oxygen atoms can become unpaired and unstable, forming free radicals.

FREE RADICALS AND OXIDATION

Oxygen is only one source of free radicals. Oxidation occurs naturally in the body in many different processes, or it can come from external sources, such as exposure to radiation, heavy metals, or synthetic chemicals. If your body is damaged by free radicals, it is less able to control the aging process and to prevent the risk factors for the formation of tumors and cancers, hardening of the arteries, degenerative joint diseases, and many other degenerative conditions.

A basic understanding of science is needed to truly comprehend free radicals. Electrons are negatively charged particles that normally occur in stable pairs. A free radical is an unstable atom that has an unpaired electron available to bond with other atoms or molecules. When an unpaired electron (free radical) bonds with the substances that make up the body's tissues, it can cause oxidative damage. Free radicals create four primary substances as byproducts of various metabolic processes within the body: hydrogen peroxide, hydroxyl, lipid peroxide, and superoxide.

Each free radical is capable of destroying an entire enzyme or protein, even an entire cell. Through a process called *biological magnification,* a few free radicals can cause a chain reaction, creating thousands of destructive free radicals. Oxidation is one of the greatest causes of degeneration and aging in the body.

Free radicals oxidize the cells in our bodies in six main ways. They:

1. Damage cell walls and membranes, limiting their ability to transport oxygen and nutrients into, and wastes out of, the cells.

2. Accumulate and deposit the lipofuscin (aging pigment) remaining from the destruction of damaged blood cells (lipofuscin is found in the heart and smooth muscles).

3. Cross-link DNA molecules and proteins together.

4. Damage enzymes and disrupt enzyme systems.

5. Destroy lysosomes, the digestive components of cells, causing improper digestion of other cell components.

6. Oxidize fat cells, called *lipid peroxidation,* turning them rancid.[1]

KEY POINT

Problems arise with free-radical oxidation of the body's tissues when the body produces an overabundance of free radicals or accumulates excessive free radical–causing oxidants, creating an imbalance between the number of free radicals (oxidizing agents) and anti-oxidant nutrients (reducing agents) in the body.

The sources of free radicals are many, including alcohol; tobacco; recreational and prescription drugs; hydrogenated oils; heavy-metal poisoning; pesticides; cleaning products; personal-care items; chemicals in our air, water, and food; bacteria; viruses; radiation (including sunlight); strenuous exercise; and stress. It's virtually impossible to avoid initiating and accumulating free radicals in the modern world.

However, not all free radicals are bad. Energy production depends on electron transport within the cells, which creates some free radicals. Also, your immune system creates them to kill bacteria and viruses, and the body uses them to produce certain hormones and enzymes.

ANTIOXIDANTS

An *antioxidant* decreases free-radical damage in the body. Antioxidants are found in many forms, including amino acids, herbs, minerals, vitamins, foods, and dietary supplements.

Although many antioxidants are found in foods, the chances of obtaining sufficient nutrients from eating the "standard American diet" (devitalized, packaged, processed, refined, undernutritious food, made from enzyme- and mineral-deficient, commercially grown fruits and vegetables, and loaded with extra fat, sugar, and salt) are minimal. We believe that the only way to consume enough nutrients, including antioxidants, is by supplementing the diet with high-quality nutritional supplements.

In 1967 two scientists discovered an enzyme that they determined could act as a reducing agent for a free radical known as *superoxide;* they called the enzyme *superoxide dismutase* (SOD). All cells that use oxygen to burn food and produce energy create superoxide naturally in a process called *cellular respiration.* This discovery led biochemists and physicians to research these reducing agents to see how they could help protect cells in people exposed to x-rays or radiation, both of which cause an overabundance of free radicals.

One of the most notable antioxidants tested was vitamin E. In more than thirty years of research, vitamin E has been shown to act as an antioxidant that can protect cells from free-radical damage. In the 1970s and 1980s, antioxidants including vitamins C and E were studied to determine their protective effects in various degenerative processes, including cancer and heart disease, and to address the effects of smoking tobacco. These studies came to three conclusions:

1. The antioxidants needed to counteract heart disease are more than can be easily derived from dietary sources; they must come from nutritional supplements.

2. Antioxidant nutrients can help prevent certain types of cancer.

3. People and populations who consume more antioxidants in their diets and nutritional supplements are much healthier than those who don't.

Research shows that proper antioxidant/oxidant balance in the body helps to prevent arthritis, heart disease, cancer, cataracts, and many age-related degenerative conditions. It is very difficult to obtain optimum levels of certain antioxidants from food alone.[2]

EFFECTIVENESS

Of the 75,000 chemicals registered with the Environmental Protection Agency (EPA), many are carcinogenic (cancer-causing) and many are oxidants. We literally live in a "soup" of oxidizing chemicals and metals. Although oxygen has been identified as the primary cause of free radicals, thousands of chemicals act as oxidizing agents and can initiate different forms of free radicals.

Two of the most scientifically validated antioxidant nutrients are vitamins C and E. Many people take them every day, thinking that they provide complete antioxidant protection. However, each antioxidant nutrient is a different reducing agent that may be able to quench different forms of free radicals. Consuming a variety of antioxidant-containing foods and supplements is the best way to protect the body.

Antioxidants come in both natural and synthetic forms. Three examples of synthetic antioxidants are the food preservatives butylated hydroxyanisole (BHA), butylated hydroxytoluene (BHT), and ethylenediaminetetraacetic acid (EDTA; the same substance used in chelation). Nutritional antioxidants also come in different forms: enzymes, herbs, foods, minerals, and vitamins (see Table 2.1 below).

TABLE 2.1 NUTRITIONAL ANTIOXIDANTS	
Antioxidant	**Description**
Alpha-lipoic acid	A potent antioxidant in its own right, alpha-lipoic acid recharges vitamins C and E after they have been exhausted by free radicals.
Amino acids	Cysteine, glutathione (GSH), methionine.
Carotenoids	Alpha-carotene, beta-carotene, lycopene.
Coenzyme Q_{10}	CoQ_{10} is important in cellular energy production and has numerous antiaging benefits. It is particularly helpful in cardiovascular disease and may be helpful with cancer, immune-compromised conditions, muscular conditions, diabetes, and periodontal disease.

Dietary	Cayenne pepper, garlic, turmeric.
Enzymes	Catalase, glutathione peroxidase (GPX), SOD.
Flavonoids	Also known as bioflavonoids, these antioxidants are responsible for the medicinal effect of many natural substances, including barks, flowers, fruits (especially apples, berries, citrus, and grapes), nuts, seeds, spices, teas, and vegetables.
Herbs	Astragalus, bilberry, burdock, ginkgo biloba, green tea, milk thistle, and sage.
Hormone	Melatonin.
Minerals	Copper, manganese, selenium, and zinc.
Nicotinamide adenine dinucleotide	NADH is the active coenzyme form of vitamin B_3 and is essential for cellular energy production. It is found in fish, poultry, and cattle muscle tissue and in food products made with yeast.
Oligomeric proanthocyanidins (OPCs)	Grape seed, pine bark, and Pycnogenol.
Vitamins	A, B_1, C, and E.

Antioxidants defend the cells from free-radical damage, improve the integrity and pliability of the arteries, decrease blood-cell clumping, cut LDL cholesterol levels, lessen inflammation and swelling, and reduce age-related degeneration, including arthritis, cancer, cataract formation, heart disease, and macular degeneration.

3. Chelation

The idea of using chelation to detoxify the body was first introduced in 1941. In 1948, it was used to treat workers in a battery factory for lead poisoning. Medical researchers noticed that when ethylenediaminetetraacetic acid (EDTA) was delivered intravenously, it could chelate lead from the workers' bodies. Soon afterward, the U.S. Navy advocated chelation for sailors who had been exposed to lead while painting government facilities and ships. Doctors administering intravenous (IV) EDTA chelation also noticed that patients who had atherosclerosis or arteriosclerosis experienced significant reductions in these conditions.[1] (Atherosclerosis is a progressive hardening and thickening of the walls of large and medium-sized arteries that results from fatty deposits on their inner linings. Arteriosclerosis is the hardening and thickening of arterial walls.)

Since the early 1950s, some doctors have used IV EDTA chelation to treat cardiovascular disease. How does it work? The disodium-salt portion of EDTA has a weaker molecular bond than do the minerals or metals to be chelated, that is, barium, beryllium, cadmium, calcium, chromium, cobalt, copper, lead, iron, magnesium, manganese, mercury, nickel, plutonium, strontium, or zinc. As the minerals or metals are "grabbed" by the EDTA, the weak disodium-salt bond is replaced with a new, stronger bond to the mineral or metal. This process begins to neutralize the metal's or mineral's toxic properties and prepares it for elimination.

Although most early chelation research was done with EDTA, many natural and synthetic substances can also chelate metals and minerals. Some of them act as antioxidants and support the detoxification organs, especially the liver (the primary organ that detoxifies the blood).

IV CHELATION

IV chelation therapy involves injecting a chelating agent into the blood-stream to eliminate undesirable substances, such as heavy metals, from the body. Most research has focused on lead removal.

A brief review of current prescription IV and oral chelation agents follows. You can obtain these chelating agents only with a prescription from a medical doctor. To find a doctor who provides IV chelation, contact The American College for Advancement in Medicine (949-583-7666; www.acam.org/dr_search/).

Dimercaprol

Also known as British Anti-Lewisite (BAL), dimercaprol can cross the blood-brain barrier into the central nervous system, where lead tends to accumulate. A bisulfide molecule, this fat-soluble drug must be injected into the muscles. It has the odor of sulfides (sulfur), and patients often complain of a bad taste and a variety of physical symptoms when the drug is injected.

Dimercaprol is more effective in preventing lead from accumulating than in reversing existing buildup. Adverse effects include abscess formation, fever, headache, injection-site pain, nausea, and vomiting. Dimercaprol may form toxic complexes with iron, cadmium, or selenium, and could interfere with thyroid iodine levels.

D-Penicillamine

A derivative of penicillin, D-penicillamine is approved for the treatment of Wilson's disease (excessive copper in the tissues). It has been used as an oral chelator of lead for thirty years but has never been licensed for that purpose by the Food and Drug Administration (FDA). It is effective orally and has few adverse effects. Although D-penicillamine is delivered orally, it is a prescription drug available only from a medical doctor. Don't confuse oral D-penicillamine with the oral chelation nutritional formulas discussed later.

Dimercaptosuccinic Acid (DMSA)

DMSA (aka succimer) can chelate arsenic, lead, and mercury. It is currently the only approved oral medication in the United States for children with high levels of lead in their bodies, and it is FDA-approved for the removal of mercury. Adverse effects associated with DMSA include abdominal cramps, diarrhea, flulike symptoms, headaches, hemorrhoids, loose stools, a metallic taste in the mouth, nausea, rash, and vomiting. Although DMSA is delivered orally, it is a prescription drug available only from a medical doctor. It is not an oral chelation nutritional formula.

Dimercaptopropanesulfonic Acid (DMPS)

Also known as the prescription drug Dimerval, DMPS has been used extensively in Europe for more than fifty years, but it's not yet available in the United States except under special FDA permits. Available in oral and injectable forms, DMPS has become the drug of choice for most heavy-metal poisoning in Asia and Europe. Adverse effects include fever, shivering, and skin rash. Although the FDA has not yet approved it, DMPS has been used intravenously for the removal of mercury.

Ethylenediaminetetraacetic Acid (EDTA)

The FDA approves IV chelation with EDTA, but only for lead poisoning. EDTA is not metabolized and has few toxic effects. It is water-soluble and eliminates lead via the urine. In the past thirty years, hundreds of thousands of patients have received more than 3 million IV EDTA infusions delivered by more than 1,000 medical doctors. The reported success rate for increasing blood circulation is 82 percent, provided patients receive sufficient chelation. Nearly 2,000 scientific journals have published articles regarding the use of IV EDTA chelation.[3]

In addition to the effectiveness of IV EDTA chelation therapy in treating cardiovascular disease and heavy-metal toxicity, research has documented its benefits for Alzheimer's disease, aneurysm, arthritis, autoimmune conditions, cancer, cataracts, diabetes, emphysema, gallstones, hypertension, kidney stones, Lou Gehrig's disease (amyotrophic lateral sclerosis [ALS]), osteoporosis, Parkinson's disease, scleroderma, senile dementia, stroke, varicose veins, venomous snake bite, and other conditions involving interrupted blood flow and diminished oxygen delivery.[4]

Doctors usually recommend that the following tests be performed at least once before and after a course of IV chelation therapy to establish a baseline, to monitor progress, and to rule out side effects and complications: blood pressure, blood-sugar status, cholesterol and other blood-lipid levels, kidney-function tests, liver-function tests (if there's a concern), pulse rate, and tissue-mineral and nutrient status.

Some nutritionally oriented medical doctors also provide nutrient-based IV treatments to enhance the chelation process or to address specific health conditions, including the following:

- Meyer's cocktail—a short, ten-minute IV "push" of calcium, magnesium, B vitamins (*not* including B_6 and B_{12}), vitamin C, and procaine (added to prevent pain at the infusion site).

- Magnesium infusion—helpful against asthma and migraine headaches.

- Vitamin C infusion—beneficial in fighting bacterial and viral infections and as an auxiliary therapy for cancer.[5]

- Phosphatidylcholine/glutathione infusion—useful against hepatitis C, Alzheimer's disease, Parkinson's disease, and other neurodegenerative diseases.

- Selenium/vitamin B_{12}/vitamin C infusion—valuable in treating infectious processes.

Benefits and Drawbacks

Due to its ability to remove toxic and harmful substances from the body, reduce free-radical oxidation, and improve blood flow and oxygen/nutrient delivery, EDTA is beneficial to virtually every major bodily system and helps to improve general overall health. EDTA chelates harmful heavy metals, a major source of free-radical production and oxidative damage, from the bloodstream and tissues. EDTA also takes unwanted mineral ions from the bloodstream, lowering the risk of many health conditions in which free-radical oxidation plays a part, including cancer.

As an antioxidant, EDTA decreases free-radical formation and activity in the bloodstream, diminishing oxidative damage to many crucial bodily tissues, structures, and systems; for example, enzymes, fats and oils, lipoproteins (LDL, VLDL, and HDL cholesterol), and RNA/DNA. EDTA also prevents improper calcium absorption into the cells and helps to remove unwanted calcium deposits from the arteries and tissues. And EDTA improves overall brain function, memory, concentration, and mood.

EDTA helps to restore health and flexibility to the arteries, improve cellular energy production, maintain a healthy cardiovascular system, sustain healthy cholesterol levels, and improve blood flow and oxygen delivery to the cells, tissues, muscles, organs, and glands. EDTA also reduces the "stickiness" of blood, so it's beneficial for health conditions related to blockage or narrowing of the arteries including cardiovascular disease, neurodegenerative disease, intermittent claudication, and even erectile dysfunction.

The greatest drawbacks of IV chelation therapy are the time, money, travel, and inconvenience associated with completing twenty to thirty IV chelation treatments. Relatively few doctors are trained to deliver IV chelation, so some people have to travel great distances to visit an experienced chelation doctor.

Although much safer and less expensive than coronary bypass surgery or angioplasty, IV chelation is still expensive (approximately $100 per treatment plus the charge for an office visit). IV chelation therapy infuses a large amount of EDTA directly into the bloodstream over a period of two to three hours. This sudden massive dose can be difficult for sensitive or elderly people to handle, especially if they are weak or have kidney or liver disease. And most people don't enjoy having a needle stuck in their arm for two to three hours at a time, week after week.

Many medical doctors who provide IV chelation now suggest comprehensive oral chelation formulas after a course of IV chelation to provide ongoing protection from metals, chemicals, and other toxins.

Use in Treating Coronary-Artery Disease

A retrospective study followed 470 patients with cardiovascular disease who received IV EDTA chelation therapy. The results showed marked improvements for 80 to 91 percent. Ninety-two of the 470 patients had been referred for surgical procedures, but after receiving IV EDTA chelation, only ten still needed surgery. Avoiding surgery saved an estimated $3 million in surgical and hospital fees and the up-to-six-month recovery period. The study concluded that EDTA therapy is "safe, effective, and results in cost savings."[6]

Conventional medicine treats coronary-artery disease primarily with one of three attempts to keep the artery "open":

1. Double (or more) coronary-artery bypass, which replaces blocked coronary arteries with veins taken from other areas of the body. In most cases, bypass surgery won't prolong life; however, even the most nutritionally minded cardiologists will recommend bypass surgery when it's a "quality of life" issue. When cardiovascular degeneration progresses to the point that people are experiencing an unsatisfactory quality of life, increasing blood flow surgically may be the only answer.

2. Angioplasty, which involves inserting a balloon inside a blocked artery and inflating it.

3. Stent placement, which places a stent (a rigid, hollow tube) inside a blocked artery.

All three procedures are dangerous, expensive ($25,000 to $100,000 per procedure), require a long recovery, and don't address the underlying causes of coronary-artery disease or revitalize the damaged heart and tissues.

EDTA chelation is a safe, inexpensive, and effective means of removing toxic metals from the body and revitalizing the heart. If possible, it should be considered as an alternative to surgery.

Cardiovascular revitalization is possible with the right combination of chelation, nutrition, exercise, stress reduction, and changes in diet and lifestyle. This holistic rehabilitative approach greatly reduces the cost of treatment, restores healthy heart structure and function, improves the quality of life, and extends it.[7] In most cases, IV EDTA, delivered by a licensed physician, is now considered to be an effective first alternative to surgical treatment for cardiovascular disease. So why isn't it more widely used?

According to Dr. James P. Carter, "The most frequent criticism leveled by critics of alternative medical therapies is that the new treatments are "unproven" because randomized, double-blind controlled studies have not yet been done. . . . [However,] most medical procedures routinely used . . . are also unproven using those same criteria," for example, mastectomy and prostate removal.[8] Although Dr. Carter's article was first published in 1989 and is somewhat outdated, it makes an important point.

In August 2002, the National Center for Complementary and Alternative Medicine (NCCAM) and the National Heart, Lung and Blood Institute (NHLBI), components of the National Institutes of Health (NIH), began the first large-scale clinical trial to determine the effectiveness and safety of IV EDTA chelation therapy for coronary-artery disease. The five-year study involves more than 2,300 patients at more than 100 research sites around the United States. Stephen E. Straus, M.D., NCCAM Director, stated, "The public health imperative to undertake a definitive study of chelation therapy is clear. The widespread use of chelation therapy in lieu of established therapies, the lack of adequate prior research to verify its safety and effectiveness, and the overall impact of coronary-artery disease convinced NIH that the time is right to launch this rigorous study."[9]

Many complementary and alternative medicine doctors and healthcare practitioners are skeptical that the study outcomes will reflect their ardent beliefs in the effectiveness of IV EDTA chelation for cardiovascular health. They claim that, in the past, studies involving nutritional, complementary, and alternative therapies, performed by reputable research facilities, have been carried out with ineffective protocols, or the results have been interpreted and expressed in a way that "protects the financial interests" of established medical entities. The pharmaceutical and medical industries have enormous influence in Washington.

Because these new EDTA chelation studies are being carried out by departments of the NIH, it is expected that study protocols and outcomes will be held to the highest standards. Unfortunately, health care in America is often influenced by money, politics, and the entities that are "in business with disease." To learn more about the politics of medicine and nutrition, please visit www.healthactioncenter.com/action and www.citizensforhealth.org.

ORAL CHELATION

Chelation delivered orally involves ingesting the chelating agent calcium-disodium EDTA along with other natural chelating agents. Vitamins, minerals, amino acids, antioxidants, phytonutrients, and herbs are used to supplement the benefits of the chelating agents.

EVALUATE YOUR RISK

To evaluate existing nutritional deficiencies and resulting body-chemistry imbalances, we recommend a twenty-four-hour urine analysis. This test analyzes nutritional status in general body chemistry and can determine certain organ and glandular imbalances. Data from this test can often explain why specific deficiencies and imbalances are contributing to symptoms of numerous health conditions. To evaluate levels of stored metals and chemicals in the body, we recommend hair analysis.

Simple hair analysis tests can help you determine baseline values of metals, chemicals, and other elements in your body. These tests can also show your body's ability to detoxify and protect itself.

Hair analysis is a noninvasive, accurate, and economical process of determining the body's mineral status and levels of metal toxicity. The average human scalp has about 100,000 hairs that grow about one-half inch per month. Many factors, including age, hormones, nutrition, race, and sex, affect this growth rate. As hair grows, the follicle deposits minerals and metals into the hair protein, creating a record that accurately reflects variations in mineral status and metal toxicity in body tissues.

The body stores minerals and deposits metals in the hair, nails, and teeth. By measuring hair samples, you can determine deposits and storage levels of both metals and minerals over the past two to three months. Hair analysis is considered superior to analysis of bodily fluids for three reasons:

1. The body prioritizes and maintains blood chemistry above all other body chemistries. Blood chemistry can look relatively normal, while the general body chemistry may be nutrient-deficient or dealing with a toxic load of metals and chemicals. Blood chemistry does not provide an accurate measurement of the metals and toxins being deposited and stored in body tissues and, therefore, is not a good tool for determining baseline measurements.

2. Blood analysis can measure metals and minerals only while they are in the circulating blood, before they are excreted or stored.

3. Analysis of breast milk, saliva, and urine can measure only metals and minerals excreted from the body, not those being stored.

According to the United Nations Environmental Programme, "Human hair has been selected as one of the important monitoring materials for worldwide biological monitoring."[10]

By providing a stable baseline, hair analysis lets you and your healthcare professional create a diet, detoxification program, and mineral/nutritional program specific to your body's needs. Periodic retesting of the hair accurately measures the progress of IV or oral chelation treatments, detoxification programs, or therapeutic mineral and nutrient programs. It can also show changes in metal or mineral levels due to dietary changes. If a health problem occurs, testing can identify where to apply corrective measures, hopefully before symptoms progress into a full-blown disease state.

Hair analysis for heavy metals can determine a baseline value of accumulated metals, such as aluminum, arsenic, cadmium, copper, lead, mercury, and nickel, and can determine whether heavy-metal accumulation and toxicity might be contributing to your health condition.

Shortcomings in the accuracy of hair analysis have certainly occurred in the past. However, healthcare practitioners who use hair analysis as a diagnostic tool today feel that it is valuable for determining a baseline measurement to compare to a future hair analysis to determine the success of a detoxification therapy. The purpose is to gain a "snapshot" of recent deposits of minerals and metals from which to formulate a treatment plan. It's that simple.

Some say that hair analysis is an imperfect diagnostic tool and call for standardization of values for mineral elements found within hair. However, this is nearly impossible, as no two people are exactly alike in their biochemistry, nutritional status, or hair-mineral status. (Appendix A contains a list of some laboratories that provide hair analysis tests for healthcare professionals.)

Each person is unique in his or her genetics, biochemistry, nutritional status, degree of degeneration, and physiological ability to heal, repair, and regenerate. To set goals for oral chelation and nutritional therapy, first visit a medical doctor to evaluate your cardiovascular health status with traditional diagnostic tests. Then, seek out a nutrition-oriented medical doctor or qualified health professional (doctor of naturopathic medicine, nutrition-oriented doctor of chiropractic, or qualified nutrition consultant) to obtain an analysis of your hair and/or urine to establish baseline data for heavy-metal and toxic-element status, antioxidant status, and tissue vitamin and mineral levels (see "Evaluate Your Risk" on page 28).

The biochemical processes involved in oral chelation and comprehensive nutrition are complex. Simply put, they safely remove heavy metals and undesirable minerals involved in free-radical formation, improper blood clotting, and arterial plaque formation—the underlying cause of arteriosclerosis. Many advanced oral chelation formulas contain multiple vitamins and minerals, plus proven nutritional ingredients that protect, maintain, support, and enhance the tissues, glands, organs, and body systems—readily available, safe, effective, "targeted" therapeutic formulas that are appropriate for most Americans. (For a list of companies providing oral chelation formulas, see Appendix B.)

THE EDTA CONTROVERSY

Oral calcium-disodium EDTA chelation has all the benefits of IV chelation but is much slower to act because only about 5 percent of an oral EDTA dose is absorbed from the intestines into the bloodstream, versus 100 percent from an IV EDTA infusion.[11] Taken on a daily basis over a few months, oral chelation will gradually accomplish what its IV counterpart does in a few administrations.

A combined oral chelation and targeted nutritional formula approach has numerous advantages and benefits over IV EDTA chelation alone. This type of comprehensive oral chelation formula can simultaneously address many of the underlying causes of common degenerative diseases and specifically support the involved cells, tissues, glands, organs, and body systems. Oral chelation helps to reduce heavy-metal toxicity and calcification, lower blood cholesterol, lessen the free-radical oxidation of metabolized fats, thin the blood, and reduce the formation of blood clots.

Calcium-disodium EDTA is a safe and effective blood thinner. Chronic aspirin use, on the other hand, is known to cause gastric bleeding. And the popular prescription blood thinner, Coumadin, is listed in California Proposition 65 (Clean Water Act) as a known carcinogen. Current Coumadin users can find this warning on the product information sheet that comes with the prescription.[12]

Although only about 5 percent of the EDTA consumed orally passes into general circulation; it binds with consumed toxic metals in the stomach and intestines, preventing their absorption into the bloodstream. Also, EDTA prevents the reabsorption of metals carried in the bile from the liver and gallbladder into the intestinal tract.

Some detractors of oral chelation therapies caution that the 95 percent of the EDTA that is undigested blocks the absorption of many healthy metals and minerals. For this reason, those who consume EDTA orally should also take a daily vitamin/mineral/antioxidant formula, which replaces any "good" minerals and metals lost in the chelation process.

EDTA is a powerful antioxidant. It helps reduce the oxidation of bile and numerous other intestinal substances, lowering the risk of colon cancer.

Adding nutrients known to support liver function and detoxification increases the effectiveness of a combination oral chelation and

KEY POINT

The heightened benefits of oral chelation over IV EDTA chelation result from the synergistic effect of combining calcium-disodium EDTA with nutrients known to support the cleansing and tissue nourishment processes. These nutrients include activated clays, bioflavonoids, chlorella, cilantro, coenzyme Q_{10}, garlic, L-cysteine, L-glutathione, lipoic acid, methionine, selenium, and zinc. Current studies indicate that oral chelation formulas have the ability to chemically bond with and eliminate aluminum, arsenic, cadmium, lead, mercury, and nickel from the body.[13]

nutrition formula. A companion formula of antioxidants and other nutrients can enhance the process by replacing any beneficial minerals and metals removed during chelation, promoting tissue healing, and preventing further free-radical oxidative damage. A variety of antioxidant nutrients can quench free radicals, so companion formulas should contain a broad spectrum of them.

Many leading physicians and scientists believe that free radicals are a primary factor in virtually all degenerative disease states. Using various antioxidant nutritional supplements in addition to EDTA may be one reason that combination formulas are so successful.

We should all review our lifestyles to see how they are affecting our health. All are encouraged to adopt healthier ways of living, including reducing or eliminating tobacco smoke, eating healthy foods, maintaining a healthy weight, exercising regularly, and reducing stress to enhance the overall healing process. But regardless of lifestyle changes, chelation has been scientifically proven to work.

4. IV & Oral Chelators and Supportive Nutrients

The nutrients to look for in a comprehensive oral chelation formula include, but are not limited to: natural chelating agents (nutrients that assist in the mobilization of metals and toxins); amino acids; antioxidants; minerals; vitamins; lipotrophic nutrients, which assist in the breakdown of fats and fatty deposits; nutrients that support liver function and the body's detoxification pathways; phyto- (plant-based) nutrients that support the structure and function of the heart and vascular system; and plant-based enzymes. Some of these substances have the ability to pass through the blood-brain barrier and mobilize heavy metals from the brain and nerve ganglions or provide antioxidant, free-radical scavenging effects in the central nervous system.

1. ALPHA-LIPOIC ACID

A vitaminlike substance, alpha-lipoic acid is a powerful antioxidant with the unique ability to protect the body from both fat-soluble and water-soluble oxidative free radicals. It helps to treat a number of liver-related conditions including those caused by carbon-tetrachloride, metal, and mushroom poisoning, alcohol-caused liver damage, and diabetic polyneuropathy. Alpha-lipoic acid is a companion to lead chelation, because it can decrease oxidative stress and protect cell membranes.

2. ARTICHOKE

This leaf extract stimulates bile production in the liver and increased bile release from the gallbladder. It helps to eliminate toxic substances from the bloodstream, normalize blood-cholesterol levels, and lower blood lipids, and it provides liver-protective qualities.

3. BIOFLAVONOIDS

These antioxidants are a class of water-soluble plant pigments that have anti-inflammatory, antihistaminic, and antiviral properties. They can chelate metals, particularly iron, protect vitamin C, decrease capillary fragility, and help to prevent blood clots. Bioflavonoids scavenge oxidative free radicals, and protect red blood cells from exposure to silica and asbestos.

Flavonoids include catechin, cynarin, hesperidin, quercetin, rutin, and silymarin. A recent study showed that people with higher flavonoid intake had a lower mortality from ischemic heart disease and cerebrovascular disease, and a lower incidence of asthma, lung cancer, prostate cancer, and type 2 diabetes.

4. BIOTIN

Biotin is a water-soluble vitamin, classified as a B-complex vitamin. This vitamin regulates energy and promotes strong nails and healthy hair and skin. It is also needed to break down and utilize fatty acids, manufacture and use amino acids (proteins), and utilize glucose and the B vitamins.

5. CALCIUM

Essential for the formation and repair of your bones, teeth, and nails, sufficient calcium helps to prevent bone loss and reduces the risk of osteoporosis. It also plays a role in blood clotting, cell-membrane function, maintenance of healthy blood pressure, proper muscle contraction, proper nerve transmission, regulation of the heartbeat, and release of neurotransmitters.

In people with excessive cholesterol levels, this mineral decreases LDL levels and increases HDL levels. Low calcium levels are directly associated with elevated C-reactive protein levels, which are found with increased inflammation and more cardiac and vascular "events." It also helps prevent cardiovascular disease and cancer and reverse fluorosis. As an oral chelate, calcium displaces toxic metals from the body. It also helps to prevent cardiovascular disease and cancer and to reverse fluorosis. And it protects the bones and teeth from lead by inhibiting lead absorption.

6. CHLORELLA

A fresh-water algae, chlorella is a good source of chlorophyll, which can help to cleanse the blood of toxins and protect the body from the effects of ultraviolet radiation. Chlorophyll can prevent the absorption of seven types of dioxin-based chemicals and ten types of polychlorinated diben-zofuran, when these chemicals are ingested with food.

Chlorella promotes the elimination of numerous metals from the body, including cadmium, chromium, copper, lead, manganese, nickel, and zinc. The algae cell wall can absorb toxic metals and enable the mobilization of mercury from within the cell, brain, and central nervous system. High doses of chlorella appear to be very effective for mercury elimination.

7. CHOLINE

This member of the B-vitamin family is important for proper liver function and to reduce the incidence of certain cancers. Choline is used to treat chronic hepatitis (inflammation of the liver), cirrhosis (fibrotic inflammatory disease of the liver), dementia, high cholesterol, liver disease, memory loss, and Parkinson's disease.

Choline is needed for the proper transmission of nerve impulses from the brain throughout the central nervous system, for gallbladder regulation, and for proper liver function. It helps to produce hormones, metabolize fat and cholesterol, and minimize excess fatty deposits in the liver. A deficiency in choline may also result in cardiac symptoms, high blood pressure, and the inability to digest fats.

8. CHONDROITIN SULFATE

This nutrient is a constituent of the arterial wall and possesses natural anticoagulant and anti-inflammatory properties.

9. CILANTRO

Also called Chinese parsley, this extract can rapidly mobilize aluminum, lead, mercury, and tin from the brain and central nervous system. The mobilized mercury appears to be either excreted via the stool or urine, or moved to more peripheral tissues. Cilantro alone often does not remove mercury from the body; it only displaces the metals from inside the cell or from deeper body stores to more peripheral tissues, where they can be more easily removed by intravenous (IV) or oral chelation therapies. The use of cilantro with dimercaptosuccinic acid (DMSA) or dimercapto-propanesulfonic acid (DMPS) has produced an increase in motor nerve function. Although cilantro alone doesn't remove mercury from the body, it is the first natural substance known to mobilize mercury from the central nervous system.

10. COENZYME Q_{10}

CoQ_{10} is produced by the liver and can be obtained from some dietary sources; however, as you age, your body's ability to produce CoQ_{10} diminishes. Remember, your heart is a pump that must never stop. The primary cellular energy-production process in your body depends upon the presence of CoQ_{10}. The organs that naturally contain the highest levels of CoQ_{10} are the heart, kidneys, liver, and muscles. Factors that impair optimal CoQ_{10} production by the liver include aging, liver damage (even mild cases), low-protein or strict vegetarian diets, genetic abnormalities, and disease states such as coronary heart disease and immune suppression).

Oral supplementation with CoQ_{10} has been shown to support the healthy functioning of the heart, improve energy levels, and improve immune-system function. Numerous studies have documented that people suffering from different forms of cardiovascular disease are often deficient in CoQ_{10}. Significant clinical improvement has been reported when supplemental CoQ_{10} has been added to conventional therapies for heart disease. Disease states associated with CoQ_{10} deficiencies include angina, congestive heart conditions, coronary heart disease, gingivitis, hypertension (high blood pressure), immune-system dysfunction, periodontal disease, and premature aging. The combination of CoQ_{10} and L-carnitine may be the most beneficial nutrients for supporting and maintaining proper cardiovascular health and energy production.

Certain prescription drugs, including statin drugs used to lower cholesterol, antidepressant drugs, and antihypertensive drugs used to lower blood pressure, are known to decrease CoQ_{10} production by the body. People who consume these drugs should supplement with CoQ_{10}

However, not all CoQ_{10} products are created equal. CoQ_{10} has a large particle size and is not usually absorbed well into the bloodstream. Look for "hydrosoluble" CoQ_{10}, or look for companies that offer "improved absorption and bioavailability."

11. ENZYMES

These biological catalysts are the primary motivators of all life processes in the body. Current research examines the effectiveness of the plant enzymes protease, lipase, carbohydrase, and cellulase preparations in controlled studies in a wide range of conditions including indigestion, malabsorption, celiac disease, and arterial obstruction. The enzymes lipase, catalase, and superoxide dismutase (SOD) are very important to break down fats and protect the body from free-radical oxidation.

Lipase, a lipotrophic agent, aids in fat digestion by hydrolyzing fat, yielding fatty acids and glycerol.

Catalase, one of the most potent antioxidant enzymes, has the ability to neutralize hydrogen peroxide and liberate useful oxygen for the body. The brain uses three main enzymes to guard against free radicals. These three enzymes are catalase, SOD, and glutathione peroxidase (GPX).

Superoxide dismutase (SOD) protects cells and tissues from oxygen-caused free-radical damage. Our bodies cannot manufacture SOD; it must be obtained from the diet or dietary supplements. A potent antioxidant, this enzyme helps to transform the highly toxic superoxide free radical into oxygen and hydrogen peroxide. SOD also counteracts inflammation and protects against cataract formation.

12. EVENING PRIMROSE OIL (EPO)

EPO naturally contains 2 to 16 percent gamma-linolenic acid (GLA) and 65 to 80 percent linoleic acid. EPO possesses anti-inflammatory properties, making it beneficial for cardiovascular disease, dermatitis and eczema, premenstrual syndrome, rheumatoid arthritis, and numerous other inflammation-related conditions.

13. FLAXSEED OIL

Flaxseed oil naturally contains linolenic, linoleic, and oleic acids and is a good source of alpha-linolenic acid, which increases serum omega-3 fatty acid levels. Alpha-linolenic acid is necessary for the healthy structure and functioning of cells. Flaxseed oil includes eicosapentaenoic acid (EPA) and docosahexaenoic acid (DHA).

Flaxseed oil supports cardiovascular health by decreasing blood-platelet clumping, increasing arterial elasticity, improving circulation, lowering LDL cholesterol and triglyceride levels, providing natural anti-inflammatory effects, and reducing atherosclerosis (hardening of the arteries due to fatty deposits).

14. FISH OIL

Daily supplementation with omega-3 fatty acids is recommended due to low dietary intake of this "healthy" fat. Omega-3s are found in high quantities in fish, including cod, halibut, herring, mackerel, salmon, and tuna. Fish oils include EPA and DHA, which possess health benefits including anti-inflammatory properties, slowing the proliferation of tumor cells, reducing the risk of cardiovascular disease and mortality, lowering the levels of LDL cholesterol and triglycerides, and decreasing blood pressure.

Since 1950, many foods and infant formulas have been sold that lack DHA and other omega-3 fatty acids. DHA deficiency is associated with increased levels of aggressive hostility, attention deficit hyperactivity disorder (ADHD), cystic fibrosis, depression, and fetal alcohol syndrome. DHA is recommended for adult-onset diabetes, arthritis, atherosclerosis, some cancers, depression, heart attacks, and high blood pressure.

15. FOLIC ACID

This nutrient (with B_6 and B_{12}) is necessary to sustain healthy homocysteine levels, maintain heart health, create DNA, form hemoglobin in red blood cells, and reduce the risk of neural-tube birth defects. It is important not to megadose with this nutrient during the chelation process.

16. GARLIC

This root herb lowers LDL cholesterol, triglycerides, and total blood-cholesterol levels, and is used to prevent arteriosclerosis (hardening and thickening of the artery walls), high blood pressure, and cardiovascular disease. It offers a protective effect for the elastic properties of the aorta in elderly people and has been shown to reduce blood-platelet aggregation. Garlic also imparts a protective effect against and increases the excretion of cadmium, lead, and mercury.

Allicin, the active ingredient in garlic, has a variety of antimicrobial properties. It provides antibacterial activity against gram-negative and gram-positive bacteria, including multidrug-resistant strains of *E. coli;* antifungal activity, particularly against *Candida albicans;* antiparasitic activity, including some major human intestinal protozoan parasites, such as *Entamoeba histolytica* and *Giardia lamblia;* and antiviral activity.

17. GINKGO BILOBA

This powerful herbal antioxidant improves blood flow to the brain, particularly in older people whose blood vessels have been narrowed and hardened by atherosclerosis or arteriosclerosis. It also helps improve the use of oxygen and glucose in the brain.

Ginkgo biloba shows promise in the treatment of neurological symptoms associated with Alzheimer's disease, brain injury, edema, normal aging, ringing in the ears, and stroke. Ginkgo may also have a role in improving memory and cognitive speed, handling activities of daily living (ADL), treating edema, lessening inflammation, and dealing with free-radical toxicity.

Although ginkgo has very few side effects or drug interactions, it does thin the blood. Caution is advised if people already take aspirin daily as a blood thinner or take an anticoagulant (blood-thinning) drug, such as Coumadin.

18. GLUTATHIONE (GSH)

GSH is a powerful antioxidant that is synthesized in the liver from cysteine, glutamic acid, and glycine. It helps the liver to cleanse harmful toxins and environmental poisons. GSH promotes protection from oxidizing free radicals, chemical pollution, carcinogens, toxins, and radiation damage, as well as recovery from burns and surgery and detoxification of metals and prescription (and OTC) drugs. GSH is also important in the formation of proteins, prostaglandins, and DNA and in the maintenance of DNA. It's a factor in the function and maintenance of the immune system and the activation of certain enzymes.

We now suspect that a combination of oxidative stress and diminished GSH status are common underlying risk factors for Lou Gehrig's disease, Parkinson's disease, and Alzheimer's disease. As its levels in human plasma decrease with age, numerous degenerative processes, including macular degeneration and diabetes, increase. In addition, there is a direct relationship between GSH levels in the body and the incidence of gastrointestinal cancers and other diseases of the gastrointestinal tract.

19. HAWTHORN BERRY

This extract is nutritional support for various cardiovascular conditions. It can increase the integrity of the blood-vessel wall, improve coronary blood flow, provide positive effects on oxygen utilization, and have a beneficial effect on blood lipids.

20. L-CARNITINE

Similar in structure to an amino acid, L-carnitine is actually related to a B vitamin. Its main function is to shuttle dietary fats (long-chain fatty acids) to each cell's mitochondria, where they are used as fuel for energy production. L-carnitine is crucial for energy production in the muscles and heart. Patients with congestive heart failure often have an L-carnitine deficiency.

L-carnitine is used to treat numerous kinds of chronic liver disease. It increases exercise tolerance, even in cardiovascular patients with ischemia or "effort-induced" angina. It has also been used successfully to fight chronic fatigue syndrome. The combination of L-carnitine and CoQ_{10} is very beneficial for cardiovascular health, energy production, and immune-system health.

21. L-CYSTEINE

This amino acid and antioxidant protects the body from free-radical oxidation. L-cysteine protects against oxidizing free radicals, chemicals, and toxins. It reduces the effects of aging and is used in protein formation and burn treatment, and for recovery from surgery. A part of proper immune-system function, L-cysteine also helps to maintain elastin production and skin health.

22. L-LYSINE

This amino acid is required for the creation and repair of collagen. L-lysine helps to repair the structure of damaged collagen in arteriosclerotic blood vessels. Primarily used to suppress the herpes simplex virus, L-lysine is also therapeutic for cardiovascular disease and osteoporosis. It enhances intestinal calcium absorption and improves the kidney's ability to conserve absorbed calcium. L-lysine supplements are recommended both preventively and therapeutically for osteoporosis.

23. L-METHIONINE

An essential, sulfur-containing amino acid, L-methionine helps remove heavy metals from the body and protects against the toxic effects of radiation. L-methionine chelates lead and is effective in preventing liver damage, including acetaminophen poisoning, and supporting liver function. L-methionine is a powerful antioxidant that also helps people with chemical allergies. It assists in the breakdown of fat, and helps prevent fatty buildup in the liver and arteries.

This amino acid promotes the excretion of estrogen and helps to detoxify xenobiotics, which are estrogenlike, nonpolar, fat-soluble, environmental chemical substances that can interfere with normal estrogen functions and fertility and contribute to cancer formation in both humans and animals.

24. LYCOPENE

This carotenoid gives tomatoes their red color. Lycopene is an antioxidant that provides protection from free-radical tissue damage, reduces the risk of cardiovascular disease and cancer—especially lung, prostate, and stomach cancers.

25. MAGNESIUM

This mineral plays an important role in the formation of bones and teeth. It is involved in energy production, where it acts as a catalyst for numerous enzymatic reactions. Magnesium helps to regulate calcium metabolism and the secretion and action of insulin. It is crucial for proper muscle control and relaxation (as in Epsom salts), and for nerve and cardiac function. It displaces toxic metals including arsenic, cadmium, and lead. Magnesium, calcium, and potassium play a significant role in the regulation of healthy blood-pressure levels.

Magnesium is very important for anyone with cardiovascular disease. Magnesium deficiency is associated with atherosclerosis, cardiac arrhythmias, congestive heart failure, ischemic heart disease, progressive vasoconstriction of the coronary vessels, sudden cardiac death, and ventricular complications from diabetes mellitus, as well as renal (kidney) disease, neuromuscular conditions and neuropathy, premenstrual syndrome (PMS), and adult-onset diabetes. Combining magnesium and CoQ_{10} reduces many symptoms of heart disease, including chest pain, easy fatigability, palpitations, and shortness of breath.

26. METHYLSULFONYLMETHANE (MSM)

MSM is a good source of sulfur, which the body uses to create glutathione (GSH), taurine, and N-acetylcysteine (NAC), important nutrients used by the liver in the detoxification process. MSM has been shown in studies to be effective for the treatment of allergies, athletic injuries, and pain syndromes.

27. N-ACETYLCYSTEINE (NAC)

The acetylated variant of L-cysteine, NAC is a chelating agent used to treat acute heavy-metal poisoning and adverse reactions to chemical drugs. It helps to protect the liver and kidneys from damage, and it enhances the elimination of metals from the body.

NAC contains sulfur and supports Phase II of liver detoxification through the process of sulfanation. Its free-radical reducing properties are useful in treating pulmonary disease and cardiovascular disease, thereby preventing heart attacks. NAC has natural anti-inflammatory properties and can reduce cellular production of numerous "pro-inflammatory mediators," such as tumor necrosis factor–alpha and interleukin. NAC is an effective antidote in acetaminophen poisoning. It has been used in clinical practice for more than thirty years.

28. OLIGOMERIC PROANTHOCYANIDINS (OPCS)

OPCs are highly bioavailable antioxidants that improve circulation and help to maintain the health of blood vessels and the heart. OPCs are extracted from numerous natural substances, including grape seeds, peanut skins, and pine-tree bark, and contain beneficial bioflavonoids. The name "Pycnogenol" was originally intended to describe all products containing procyanidins. Presently, Pycnogenol products containing extracts from French maritime pine bark are marketed under the registered trademark of Horphage Research Ltd. OPCs are potent scavengers of free radicals, especially ascorbyl and tocopheryl radicals, thus helping to maintain levels of vitamins C and E. OPCs are also powerful, natural anti-inflammatory agents and thus help to protect body organs from drug or chemical-induced toxicity; to protect against ultraviolet radiation; to improve lung function in asthmatics; to modulate the immune system; to reduce platelet stickiness; and to improve cognitive functions.

29. PHYTOSTEROLS

These plant fats play a role in plants similar to that of cholesterol in humans, primarily in forming cell-membrane structures, sources of fuel for storage and transport, and protective surface coatings. The most common plant sterols are beta-sitosterol, campesterol, and stigmasterol. Phytosterols have antihyperglycemic and insulin-releasing effects, anti-inflammatory and antipyretic activities, and immune-regulating activities, which may be beneficial for allergies, autoimmune diseases, cancer, chronic viral infections, rheumatoid arthritis, and tuberculosis. Phytosterols lower LDL and total cholesterol levels without affecting HDL cholesterol levels, decreasing the risk of cardiovascular disease.

30. POTASSIUM

This mineral helps to maintain fluid levels in your body. It is essential for the conversion of blood sugar into glycogen, which exercising muscles use for energy and for kidney and adrenal function. Potassium is important in numerous biochemical functions, including acid-base (pH) balance, cellular electrochemical processes, enzyme reactions, blood-pressure regulation, and proper heart rhythm, muscle contractions, nerve conduction, and gastric-fluid secretion.

31. RED RICE YEAST

This nutrient is produced from a specific strain of yeast and prepared by a rice fermentation process. Red yeast is recommended to lower LDL cholesterol levels, decrease total cholesterol levels, and reduce triglyceride levels.

32. SELENIUM

Fundamentally important for human health, this mineral is a key element in preventing coronary disease and is a part of the body's antioxidant arsenal. Selenium is the biological catalyst for the production of active thyroid hormone. It supports proper immune function, reducing the risk of cancer and other immune-related conditions, and has a protective effect against diabetic complications of cardiovascular disease. Selenium also helps to prevent toxic reactions to mercury.

33. TRIMETHYLGLYCINE (TMG)

TMG (also called glycine betaine or betaine anhydrous) is a natural methyl-group donor. Excessive homocysteine levels are associated with cardiovascular disease. Methylating factors (substances that donate methyl groups causing the conversion of unhealthy homocysteine into the nontoxic amino acid methionine) can reduce levels of homocysteine. Vitamins B_6, B_{12}, and folic acid are often recommended for maintaining healthy homocysteine levels; however, if those vitamins don't work, TMG can be used. It is a lipotrophic nutrient and assists in fat metabolism. Due to its beneficial effects on oxidative stress and insulin sensitivity, TMG is useful against nonalcoholic fatty-liver disease. The use of methyl-group donors to maintain healthy homocysteine levels is important for supporting cardiovascular health. Some concern has been raised regarding the potential for converting elemental mercury into the more toxic methylmercury when methyl-group donor nutrients are used during the chelation process. Research shows that this is possible if megadosing with vitamins B_6, B_{12}, folic acid, and TMG.[1]

34. VITAMIN A

This vitamin is necessary for the development of healthy bones and teeth, the growth and repair of body tissues, a healthy immune system, healthy skin and hair, night vision, and reproduction.

35. VITAMIN B₁ (THIAMINE)

Thiamine is necessary for antioxidant protection, converting carbohydrates into glucose to produce energy, forming blood cells, proper metabolism of fats and proteins, healthy brain function, healthy nervous-system function, and proper muscle function, especially of the heart muscle.

36. VITAMIN B₂ (RIBOFLAVIN)

Riboflavin is necessary to break down, utilize, and metabolize carbohydrates, fats, and proteins; produce energy; create healthy skin, hair, and nails; maintain healthy vision; provide healthy nervous-system function; and properly form red blood cells.

37. VITAMIN B₃ (NIACIN)

Niacin is necessary for energy production; metabolism and utilization of carbohydrates, fats, and proteins; proper nervous-system function; blood-sugar regulation; and blood-vessel dilation (widening blood vessels and increasing blood flow).

38. VITAMIN B₅ (PANTOTHENIC ACID)

Pantothenic acid is necessary to release energy from carbohydrates, fats, and proteins; to manufacture adrenal hormones and red blood cells; and to form fatty acids.

39. VITAMIN B₆ (PYRIDOXINE)

Pyridoxine is necessary to maintain healthy homocysteine levels, promote heart health, metabolize proteins, create red and white blood cells, and produce neurotransmitters. It's important not to megadose with this nutrient during the chelation process.

40. VITAMIN B$_{12}$ (CYANOCOBALAMIN)

Cyanocobalamin is necessary for utilizing fatty acids for energy, maintaining healthy homocysteine levels, providing heart health, creating DNA, producing red blood cells, and producing proper folic-acid metabolism, immune-system function, and nervous-system function. It is important not to megadose with this nutrient during the chelation process.

41. VITAMIN C

Oxidative damage causes many degenerative diseases. Vitamin C, one of the most important antioxidants, easily crosses the blood-brain barrier and reaches the brain cells where it protects the brain, lowers the risk of dementia and stroke, and improves cognitive function. It can slow the progression of hardening of the carotid artery. High intakes of vitamin C lower the risk of a number of chronic diseases, including cancer, eye disease, heart disease, and neurodegenerative conditions. Vitamin C is helpful for people suffering from heart failure because it increases the availability of nitric oxide.

Vitamin C also helps to maintain healthy blood-pressure levels, supports healthy immune function, and reduces cold and flu symptoms. It supports healthy cholesterol levels and has clot-dissolving properties, promoting arterial health. It can inhibit platelet clumping, increase clot-dissolving activity, and increase HDL cholesterol values.

This vitamin has detoxifying actions on lead, mercury, carbon monoxide, sulfur dioxide, various carcinogens, bacterial toxins, and poisons; and it protects us from benzene exposure. It is a very effective detoxifier of heavy metals and chemical poisons. In addition, vitamin C supplements reduce the skin damage caused by ultraviolet light.

42. VITAMIN D

This vitamin is necessary for proper absorption and utilization of calcium and phosphorus, for proper growth and development, and for healthy bones, teeth, and nails.

43. VITAMIN E

Tocopherols and tocotrienols are necessary for antioxidant protection, preventing cell-membrane damage, improving blood circulation, inhibiting the oxidation of LDL cholesterol, maintaining heart health, promoting healthy immune function, providing healthy nerve function, sustaining heart-muscle function, protecting red blood cells, and strengthening capillary walls.

44. ZINC

An essential mineral element, zinc is the second most abundant trace mineral in the body. It acts as a cofactor in numerous biochemical processes, including the formation of DNA, RNA, and protein. More than 300 different enzymes contain zinc, and almost 100 of them use zinc in their catalytic activity. This mineral plays a part in behavior and learning ability, blood clotting, growth and development, immune function, insulin action and metabolism, reproduction, taste and smell, thyroid-hormone function, and wound healing.

5. Who Benefits?

Virtually everyone who lives in the modern world can benefit from an intravenous (IV) or oral chelation detoxification program. The most common causes of death in America are heart disease, cancer, stroke, chronic obstructive pulmonary disease (COPD), accidents and injuries, diabetes, influenza and pneumonia, Alzheimer's disease, and kidney disease.[1] All causes except accidents and injuries, influenza and pneumonia, suicide, and infant death are connected to reduced circulation of blood, nutrients, and oxygen to the tissues.

Those who receive the greatest benefits from oral chelation and nutrition therapy are those who:

- Have a family history of or have been diagnosed with a degenerative disease.

- Want to preserve, maintain, support, and enhance their health, energy, and vitality.

- Eat the standard American diet.

- Are regularly exposed to synthetic chemicals by consuming alcohol, tobacco, or drugs (prescription or recreational); by using chemical-based personal-care products (hair, skin, and body products); living in homes or working in offices made of synthetic materials; using commercial cleaning products; working with or living around synthetic chemicals (paints, smokes, fumes, solvents, cleaners, fertilizers, herbicides, pesticides, and other -cide products); drinking or bathing in tap water; driving in commuter traffic (breathing exhaust fumes); and frequently using or abusing harmful substances.

What we have seen over and over again with thousands of clients is that if you can achieve some or all of the following steps, you can dramatically improve your health condition, prevent future disease, and have the best chance of maintaining and protecting your health. These steps are to:

1. Create nutritional sufficiency where there is deficiency.

2. Create digestive competence with targeted digestive-enzyme therapy.

3. Balance body chemistry by nutritionally supporting the structure and function of involved tissues, glands, and organs with targeted nutritional therapies.

4. Gently detoxify your body daily with an IV or oral chelation program and nutritional liver support, once your body is nutritionally sufficient and has an energy reserve.

5. Modify your diet and pay attention to how your body feels one-half to one hour after eating.

6. Start drinking sufficient filtered water, using this formula: Divide your body weight by two. This equals the number of ounces of filtered water you should drink every day.

7. Create programs for regular exercise (at least twenty minutes, three times per week) and stress reduction (dancing, playing, exercising, hobbies, and so on).

8. Reduce (or seek professional help for) bad habits and addictions.

A multitude of "roadblocks" prevent the expression of vibrant health in the human body. The biggest roadblocks are nutritional deficiencies, resulting body-chemistry imbalances, accumulated chemical and metal toxins, and stress. Once these roadblocks are removed or broken through and a customized therapeutic program is instituted, a person's health changes for the better.

Recovering health using a holistic program works by natural law. It's like a mathematical equation: When you change the numbers on one side of the equal sign, the numbers on the other side will change. When you use IV or oral chelation to remove chemicals and metals from your body, the treatment diminishes the toxic load that your body must eliminate daily, improves your body chemistry and nutritional status, and allows your whole body to express health and well-being. When applied correctly, nutrition and oral chelation therapy work safely and effectively.

Recommended Laboratories

If your doctor doesn't provide hair analysis, we recommend you show him or her the following list of laboratories that provide hair analysis for licensed healthcare professionals. (For "at-home" hair and saliva analysis test kits, see Appendix C.)

Analytical Research Labs
2225 West Alice Avenue
Phoenix, AZ 85021
Phone: 602-995-1580
Fax: 602-371-8873
Website: www.arltma.com

Doctor's Data, Inc.
P.O. Box 111
West Chicago, IL 60186
Phone: 630-377-8139
Fax: 630-587-7860
Website: www.doctorsdata.com

Great Smokies Diagnostic Laboratory
63 Zillicoa Street
Asheville, NC 28801
Phone: 828-253-0621
Fax: 828-252-9303
Website: www.gsdl.com

Trace Elements
4501 Sunbelt Drive
Addison, TX 75001
Phone: 972-250-6410
Fax: 972-248-4896
Website: www.traceelements.com

APPENDIX B

Oral Chelation Formulas

Many companies market oral chelation formulas. Many are simple, often combining EDTA with one or two nutrients. Before purchasing oral chelation supplements from any manufacturer, we recommend that you thoroughly research the manufacturer. Reputable manufacturers will provide current studies, ingredient rationales, and complete product literature, if requested. The following are American manufacturers of comprehensive oral chelation supplements:

Extreme Health Inc.
2175 N. California Blvd., Suite 150
Walnut Creek, CA 94596
Fax: 925-988-8013
Toll free: 800-800-1285
Website:
    www.extremehealthusa.com
Oral chelation formulas:
Oral Chelation, Age-Less Formula

The International Institute of
    Holistic Healing
2331 Gus Thomasson, Suite 115
Dallas, TX 75228
Phone: 972-279-5525
Fax: 972-279-5525
Website: www.doctorajadams.com
Oral chelation formula:
Oral Chelation

Gordon Research Institute
708 East Highway 260, Bldg. C-1
Payson, AZ 85541
Phone: 928-472-4263
Fax: 928-474-3819
Website: www.gordonresearch.com
Oral chelation formula:
Beyond Chelation

Vibrant Life Vitamins
1831 North Bel Aire Drive
Burbank, CA 91504
Toll free: 800-523-4521
Fax: 818-558-7299
Website: www.oralchelation.com
Oral chelation formula:
Life Glow Plus

Vitamin Research Products
4610 Arrowhead Drive
Carson City, NV 89706
Toll free: 800-877-2447
Fax: 800-877-3292
Website: www.vrp.com
Oral chelation Formula:
Oral ChelatoRx 360

APPENDIX C

At-Home Laboratory Studies

BodyBalance, strategic partner of Great Smokies Diagnostic Laboratory, provides seven comprehensive at-home laboratory tests for the consumer:

1. AntiOxidantCheck monitors free-radical activity and antioxidant status.

2. FemaleCheck uses saliva to assess estradiol, progesterone, and testosterone hormone levels.

3. MaleCheck uses saliva to measure levels of testosterone and dehydroepiandrosterone (DHEA) hormones.

4. MineralCheck assesses the body's levels of eleven minerals (calcium, chromium, cobalt, copper, magnesium, manganese, molybdenum, strontium, sulfur, vanadium, and zinc) and nine toxic elements (aluminum, antimony, arsenic, bismuth, cadmium, lead, mercury, nickel, and tin).

5. PerformanceCheck measures levels of testosterone, DHEA, and cortisol hormones. Proper levels of these hormones help the body function at its maximum potential.

6. SleepCheck measures the level of melatonin hormone in the body.

7. StressCheck measures DHEA and cortisol hormone levels to determine whether they are balanced. DHEA and cortisol regulate how the body reacts during stress.

BodyBalance
63 Zillicoa Street
Asheville, NC 28801
Toll free: 888-891-3061
Fax: 828-253-4646
Website: www.bodybalance.com

Notes

Introduction

1. Wilson, C. *Chemical Exposure and Human Health* (Jefferson, NC: McFarland). 1993. pp. 1–2.

Chapter 1

1. ATSDR/EPA. "1999 Comprehensive Environmental Response, Compensation, and Liability Act (CERCLA) Priority List of Hazardous Substances." www.atsdr.cdc.gov/99list.html.

2. Schauss, A., Ph.D. *Minerals and Human Health: The Rationale for Optimal and Balanced Trace Element Levels* (Tacoma, WA: Life Sciences). 1995. pp. 4–5.

3. Pouls, M., Ph.D. "Oral Chelation and Nutritional Replacement Therapy for Chemical and Heavy Metal Toxicity and Cardiovascular Disease." *Townsend Letter for Doctors & Patients*. July 1999. pp. 82–91. Reprinted with permission.

Chapter 2

1. Passwater, R.A., Ph.D. *The Nutrition Superbook: Volume I: The Antioxidants, the Nutrients That Guard the Body against Cancer, Heart Disease, Arthritis and Allergies—and Even Slow the Aging Process* (New Canaan, CT: Keats). 1995. pp. 7–8.

2. Ibid, pp. 5–46, 329.

Chapter 3

1. Walker, M., D.P.M., and G. Gordon, M.D. *The Chelation Answer* (Atlanta, GA: Second Opinion). 1994. p. 74.

2. Walker, M., D.P.M., and H. Shah, M.D. *Everything You Should Know About Chelation Therapy* (New Canaan, CT: Keats). 1997. pp. 37–38.

3. Walker, M., D.P.M., and G. Gordon, M.D. *Ibid,* p. 14.

4. Walker, M., D.P.M. *The Chelation Way* (Garden City Park, NY: Avery). 1990. p. 54.

5. www.brightspot.org/cresearch/ivccancer.shtml.

6. Hancke, C., M.D., and K. Flytlie, M.D. "Benefits of EDTA Chelation Therapy in Atherosclerosis: A Retroactive Study of 470 Patients." *Journal of Advancement in Medicine.* 1993; 6(3):161–171.

7. Kidd, P.M. "Integrative cardiac revitalization: bypass surgery, angioplasty, and chelation. Benefits, risks, and limitations." *Alternative Medicine Review.* February, 1998; 3(1):4–17.

8. Carter, James P., M.D. "If EDTA Chelation Therapy Is So Good, Why Is It Not More Widely Accepted?" *Journal of Advancement in Medicine,* 1989; 2(1/2): 213–226.

9. http://nccam.nih.gov/news/2002/chelation/pressrelease.htm.

10. Global Environmental Monitoring System (GEMS), United Nations Environmental Programme. From the U.S. Government book *Toxic Trace Metals in Mammalian Hair and Nails* by the U.S. Environmental Protection Agency (EPA). www.traceelements.com/references.html.

11. Abraham, G., M.D. *Oral Chelation.* pp. 2–3.

12. "Oral Chelation for Improved Heart Function," Interview with Garry Gordon, M.D., D.O. www.life-enhancement.com/article_template.asp? ID=54.

13. Urinalysis studies conducted by Maile Pouls, Ph.D., and Greg Pouls, D.C., 1998. Copies of full studies available upon request from Ms. Michele Payne, President, Extreme Health Inc. Phone: 800-800-1285. www.extremehealth usa.com.

Chapter 4

1. Zorn, N.E., and J.T. Smith. "A relationship between vitamin B_{12}, folic acid, ascorbic acid, and mercury uptake and methylation." *Life Science.* 1990; 47(2):167–173.

Chapter 5

1. National Center for Chronic Disease Prevention and Health Promotion www.cdc.gov/nccdphp/overview.htm.

Index

About the Authors

Gregory Pouls, D.C., F.I.C.N., is a doctor of chiropractic, author, nutritional-product formulator, and cofounder/director of the Health Enhancement Center. For more than fifteen years, Dr. Pouls has been researching the health effects of exposure to heavy metals and synthetic chemicals and the complementary, alternative, and nutritional therapies used to reverse and overcome these conditions and prevent the future accumulation of metals and chemicals in the body.

Maile Pouls, Ph.D., is a clinical nutritionist, enzyme therapist, health educator, author, and cofounder of the Health Enhancement Center. For the past sixteen years, Dr. Pouls has been working to identify and resolve her patients' nutritional and biochemical deficiencies. Her long-distance telephone-consulting program provides individual dietary, nutritional, and detoxification protocols to support the body's natural healing abilities.

HEALTH ENHANCEMENT CENTER
866-424-HEAL (4325)
www.yournutrition.com
www.advancednutritionalconsulting.com
E-mail: drpouls@yournutrition.com

Printed in the USA
CPSIA information can be obtained
at www.ICGtesting.com
JSHW051957150824
68134JS00050B/97

9 781681 627953